OPERATION SOUL RECOVERY

(From Default To Purpose)

by
Sheryl J. Stevens

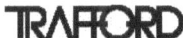

© Copyright 2005 Sheryl J. Stevens. All rights reserved.

No part of this publication may be reproduced, stored in a retrieval system, or transmitted, in any form or by any means, electronic, mechanical, photocopying, recording, or otherwise, without the written prior permission of the author.

You may contact the author at oprecovery@donobi.net

National Library of Canada Cataloguing in Publication

Stevens, Sheryl J.
    Operation soul recovery : from default to purpose / Sheryl J. Stevens ; illustrated by Alice Shull.
ISBN 1-55395-442-4
    I. Title.
RA790.S73 2003   362.2   C2002-905835-X

TRAFFORD

This book was published *on-demand* in cooperation with Trafford Publishing.
On-demand publishing is a unique process and service of making a book available for retail sale to the public taking advantage of on-demand manufacturing and Internet marketing.
On-demand publishing includes promotions, retail sales, manufacturing, order fulfilment, accounting and collecting royalties on behalf of the author.

2404 Government St., Victoria, B.C. V8T 4L7, CANADA
Phone   250-383-6864   Toll-free   1-888-232-4444 (Canada & US)
Fax   250-383-6804   E-mail   sales@trafford.com
Web site   www.trafford.com   TRAFFORD PUBLISHING IS A DIVISION OF TRAFFORD HOLDINGS LTD.
Trafford Catalogue #02-1157   www.trafford.com/robots/02-1157.html

TABLE OF CONTENTS

Introduction
Dedication
Forward
A Tribute to Heroes

PART I

Focus on the Current Problems   Page 19
of Mental Illness

PART II

The Vision for Recovery   Page 47
  (A MANOR OF EDEN)

An Overview—After 911   Page 65

PART III

About the Author   Page 73

Personal Events That Inspired the Vision   Page 75

AFTERWORD   Page 95

INTRODUCTION

The purpose of this book is unique in that it was not written just to be read. Rather, it is a compilation of many ideas and experiences of the author, directed toward a plan for a huge project that when put into action would shine a powerful light of hope in the dark corners of mental illness. A new version of the book is currently in progress, with the assistance of an editor, for expanding it into a full-length manuscript which will bring more clarity to the logic and necessity for the vision. Meanwhile, due to the time involved in completing that task, this edition is the springboard to initiate the author's compelling dream. The following 5-Star reviews are examples of responses that have been received from readers thus far:

"Sheryl Stevens writes with passion and insight about mental and emotional illness, which she is personally well acquainted with, and which is so prevalent in our society, but where treatment consists mostly of dealing with the symptoms with medication, rather than taking the harder but more constructive road to tackle the core issues that have caused the problems.

Sheryl's vision of "A Manor of Eden" is a plan to combine the spiritual and the physical, to make the person "whole", and to make them a productive part of society.

Is it feasible and is it worth a try?
The system we have in place now is spiraling out of control, and as Sheryl points out, "statistics show that the use of anti-depressants has tripled in the past decade", with little or no improvements to show for it.

Any plan that could do better than the current status quo should be given consideration, and Sheryl's plan would certainly have less recidivism than what we have now, with so many who, if they experience well-being after treatment at all, find it short-lived.

Is it too expensive ?
Not if you consider what we are paying now for a system that is not producing results, and not if you consider that if people are made well and productive, how they would enhance our economy. Sheryl's vision has a strong spiritual heart, and the acknowledgement of a Creator, something certain sectors in our society are trying to eradicate, as judges who endorse and further the agenda of radical groups make laws that are systematically tearing God out of the fabric of our lives. It is my hope that the tide of this often nihilistic secularism be stemmed, and A Manor of Eden has ideas that if implemented could help do this.

In Part III, Sheryl writes about childhood memories, of the farm she grew up on, and the boarding school she was sent to at the age of 14; we all have different sensibilities, and what was good for other family members was not good for Sheryl, and what she experienced there would influence the rest of her life in negative ways, but also surely had a hand in her vision of "A Manor of Eden", making all things ultimately work for the best. This is a small book with a lot of content, written with sincerity and conviction, with ideas that should be seriously contemplated."

- Alejandra Vernon, March 2005

"It is a little bit sad that it is not really 'news', but there is a crisis of sorts in the Western culture - America and other 'developed' nations are in fact suffering from a great number of addictions, mental illness symptoms (both real and imagined), and an ever-shrinking safety net for those least able to care for themselves.

One of the more ironic aspects of this crisis is that, in the midst of the 'lands of plenty', there would be such struggle. Even among those who fall into the affluent categories of people, depression and addiction troubles are at surprisingly high levels. What could be the cause of this? What would be the cure?

Sheryl Stevens has some suggestions. She calls for a charge against the kinds of sicknesses of the soul to be waged akin to the efforts we as a nation are putting forward in fighting the threats of terrorism. ' When it comes to diseases of the mind and spirit that inflict untold numbers of people in varying degrees on the spectrum, there is still that mysterious air of denial.' We must first face the facts of the pandemic proportions of the problems.

Stevens looks at some of the problems. She doesn't cite statistics and case studies as much as she gives a more general, thoughtful approach to the problem. What is it that we need to change? What is it that keeps us in the dark? These are key questions for Stevens, who sees real opportunities in changes of attitude and aspect for us.

Stevens has a vision, a place called 'A Manor of Eden' - taking the name from the biblical reference, this is a place where humanity is found at its most basic, and where humanity in the early stories is seen to be at its greatest possible wholeness and happiness. People who are in need of help would find those to help them, who from start to finish recognize the full humanity of each person, rather than seeing them as problems to be dealt with or case problems to be solved.

Stevens has specific proposals for residence and treatment situations for those who would find help at A Manor of Eden. She writes realistically about the cost, but also points out the tremendous costs of what are being done (often ineffectually) about the various problems in today's society.

Stevens' motivation is personal; she has encountered problems in her life, and also writes with feeling about her own upbringing, and feelings about our current situation in a post 9-11 world.

Worthy of consideration, and certainly in the same spirit as those pioneers of the American spirit who strive to make a better world for the entire community."

- Fr. Kurt Messick, April 2005

THIS BOOK IS DEDICATED TO
MY THREE CHILDREN & GRANDSON

Each one has uniquely influenced my perceptions of life and God in ways that without them, I could have never imagined. Although my spirit has been humbled by many experiences within the family, they were also the fuel that generated the passion to write this book. I now feel blessed beyond measure for the amazing gifts and lessons these children have brought into my life. Ultimately, *"With God <u>all things</u> work together for Good."*

ANOTHER DEDICATION
IS TO MY BROTHER (& only sibling)

Who passed away suddenly two weeks before Christmas 2002. Prior to his untimely death, my intention was that **he** would be the **first** recipient of the book, yet sadly did not live to see it in print. The courage to walk through these mournful shadows, will continue to be sustained by holding close the belief that he is still somewhere applauding my venture.

FOREWORD

In the absence of pain there can be no gain, nor growth of the human spirit. And what greater vulnerability do we hold than our children or grandchildren? We may be torn in every direction. The ego seeks to abandon the pain caused by the wayward child (or any family tragedy beyond our control), to at least save ourselves, or so we are apt to think. But the conscience beckons us to face this delusion, to find reason for the invasion of trials, by placing our own meager lump of clay in the Potter's hand to transform the limited thoughts. Then helplessness takes on a new meaning, *"Strength is made perfect in weakness"*. And pain, with its seasons, gently vanishes like the wind. In the magic of stillness, we begin to see the panoramic view, while hearing the beat of a different drum. The most significant change in the picture becomes its size, no longer confined to merely the eaglets in our own nest, but the vein of like malady that runs throughout other nests in the forest.

Love and Pain are the supreme motivating and creative forces on earth—the inspiration and refinement that seek to remind us *"we are spiritual beings on a human journey"*. The intended purpose of this journey is to discover the Truth about ourselves—that we are, (everyone), sons and daughters of the living God. Without this understanding, we remain lost in the wilderness of false insight and unrest, wandering in the vast range of *beautiful minds* gone awry, no matter what may be our cloak.

Within the hearts of dreamers lies the awareness that **everything** seen in the material world first began with a simple thought. Or the aphorism that, *"Any idea constantly held before the mind, MUST come into existence."* If it is one for good, then how much better to be sure of its Source. The satisfaction is in knowing that without dreams, there could never be dreams come true…

A TRIBUTE
To Heroes

The perspectives herein (taken from the storehouse of personal experience) were essentially written long before September 11th. Although partly for lack of courage in the face of rejection, they remained suspended as an unfinished substance of hope—until that jolting moment...

The alarm boldly resounded at 6:AM. It wasn't the usual blare of music, but a frantic jumble of compelling phrases shouted across the airwaves—A plane crash! The World Trade Center!... Within seconds, breaking news on the TV screen began to unfold the raging monstrosity that was taking place. Along with millions of others, I relentlessly watched and wept in horror on that dreadful day, and at the convulsing aftermath throughout the following days and weeks.

Aside from the fallen victims, we were awake, we were alive, and we were real, as we'd never been before. And somehow emerging from the grief of devastation at the most glaring example of gruesome wreckage, we began to search our own souls. Values changed in a flash. If only for a passing moment, the entire civilized world gazed in shock upon the same page. The frailty of life loomed instinctively before us—reminders of the unfulfilled dreams and hopes and unspoken words from the heart.

Was it simply a choice whether '*to be or not to be*' part of the good that would come out of this evil? Affirmatively then, it was an hour of resolve to reckon with what we, personally, had left unsaid and undone.

If there was ever a wake up call to the living, and lessons to learn, none could be more profound than the gallantry of rescue workers, the compassion and generosity of Americans across the country, the selfless heroism of military forces standing ready to defend us, or the echo of those final words by a courageous young man on Flight 93, **"*LET'S ROLL*"**... As a tribute to all victims and heroes of this disaster, **we must not forget** and fall back into the state of complacency. There is much more work to be done—never-ending challenges of enormous proportion, which can only be accomplished triumphantly in a united spirit of urgency. History has repeatedly shown us how undaunted purpose brings sustenance to the soul, just as out of the darkness of 911, patriotism was (at least) resurrected. We witnessed once again, the American valor of rising honorably to any task or crisis that comes our way.

"America, America, God shed His grace on thee. And crown thy good with brotherhood, from sea to shining sea."

"Every valley shall be exalted, every mountain and hill shall be made low, the crooked places made straight and the rough places smooth.
The glory of God shall be revealed and all people will see it together."

Is. 40:4—5

PART I

CHAPTER I

The 20th century marked America with phenomenal achievements, many of which our forefathers would have never dreamed possible. It is with great pride that most of us embrace the wonders of our heritage. Yet somewhere amidst the rush of glory over accomplishments, and bewildering controversies surrounding the rights of freedom, solid values that once guided this country seem to have fallen by the wayside. Conceivably we have arrived at the encumbering age of **information** and self-seeking passions that have managed to pale the influence of **wisdom**.

On one hand there is a growing awareness of the physical needs of people, both at home and abroad—from basic food, clothing, shelter and medicine; to preventative health measures; to abundant research in finding cures for the many dreaded diseases. Along with concerns over physical needs are those of educating the mind. Reflecting human interest, high on every politician's campaign agenda is the call for bigger and better schools, more teachers and extended learning opportunities from pre-school to college. We have seen, heard or read these ideas thousands of times throughout the media. The effect of this awareness then drives people in the quest to solve the problems. Applause toward all the achievements of betterment in human physical conditions and education resonates loud and clear.

Consequently financial support and personal involvement are readily entrusted to these worthy causes—as they rightly should be.

On the other hand, when it comes to diseases of the mind and spirit that inflict untold numbers of people in varying degrees on the spectrum, there is still that mysterious air of denial. America is respected as the most powerful world leader in nearly every arena, except genuine acknowledgement of the gravity of these problems. An alarming failure still exists in the healing of troubled souls, with widespread availability for all—a demand so great and supply so limited. Besides the suffering of those who are sick, a staggering number of other lives are also sorely affected, including the victims of their crazed behavior. Plus how many mothers especially, fathers, friends, family members, agonize every day over loved ones lost to the power of ravaging emotional disorders? According to statistics, considering our total population, **everyone** knows at least one person, if not themselves, who is stricken with an addiction or another form of mental illness. Mother Teresa so keenly once stated, *"People in countries 'round the world die of physical starvation. Americans die of emotional starvation."* The first is tragic, the second even more so...

We were horrified by the extremes of the Columbine and Oklahoma disasters, knowing that human time bombs could explode at any time in our own neighborhoods. Initially these shocking events rise to the forefront of news and discussions with conveyed emotion, then are laid to rest almost as though they never happened. The exceptions lie with the living victims who are left to grieve for a lifetime the outcomes of senseless purpose, along with the added sorrow of seeing no real lessons learned. If these kinds of atrocities alone do not evoke drastic changes in the illusive systems (presently in place) of treating mental &

emotional diseases, then it seems to be both unintelligent and confounding for a country such as ours.

The magnitude of depression with its many related forms and labels, addictions and compulsions of every sort, are all around us like plagues that sweep our land. The majority of us have learned to some extent, from early years on, that it is OK to express physical pain but not emotional pain (at least not truthfully). Nor are we taught to regard that there is no physical pain comparable to that of a broken spirit. For the most part, the needy are left to their own devices of coping in a society that continues to grow more complicated as time goes on. It's as though we have become so accustomed to the existence of these maladies that we can't see how they continue to lower the standards of our entire culture. Like *'the colossal white elephant'* in our living room we pretend not to notice. In effect we seem to be losing the very inborn sensitivity to order and decency for which we were all designed to follow.

We deny the big picture by applauding the exceptions to the rule. However deserving of attention, they are the battles won by only a scattered few. Meanwhile we have a constant multiplying number of people who are a burden and/or a threat to themselves and a civilized society. The ramifications of this unrest leave everyone else in a quandary of Fear, Anger, Frustration, Guilt, Denial, or the widespread counterbalance of Indifference. ALL OF IT creates a harmful environment for children and a toxic air for everyone to breathe. In spite of the infinite tax dollars flowing through the welfare systems; the good will and intentions of church and temple; plus all other rehabilitating efforts combined (even those that are truly wonderful)—THE JOB ISN'T GETTING DONE!

CHAPTER II

Every day thousands of severely sick people are being herded through under-staffed, poorly funded, ineffective, rehab centers with minimal individual counseling and attention. If through a government program, the patients are given three to four weeks of so-called treatment, then shipped out often to half-way houses which invariably reek with atmospheres of unmet needs. Others are recklessly turned loose with no option but returning to their negatively-charged habitats, filled with old reminders and temptations along side family and friends preoccupied with their own issues, factors that repeatedly trigger the disorders again. Although directed to continue recovery in 12-step programs, many are too vulnerable to grasp these concepts adequately, hence give up before they prove to be helpful. Reverting back to past behaviors of addiction and mental illness, cannot be simply passed off as bad choices made by weak characters, too often looked upon as the most hopeless and despised of humanity. On the contrary, they are sorely misunderstood. The minds and emotions of these people have been invaded by the most powerful forces that exist and must be appropriately treated within this mentality, until they are well and able to join society again. Little wonder that the true recovery rate has been estimated at a pitiful 5 or 6 percent at best. General opinion says, *"Its **their** fault when treatment doesn't work. They really don't want to change. Or* *if they hit bottom enough times, maybe they will...*" The effect of this nonsense is that we have 'bottomed out' people all over the place, many of whom have been through the system numerous times with little if any success, seeming a waste of everyone's time and money.

I've met many such people over the years, including one woman who was on her **22nd** round in treatment; also men and women, long-going attendants of support groups or churches who were extremely unhealthy on an emotional level. Others were as addicted to their therapists as they'd been to their drugs, over extended periods of time and making little or no headway. Or there were those, among the uncounted number, who opted to relieve their pain with prescribed medications. Some of these cases were misdiagnosed and/or left virtually unmonitored by the prescribing doctors, neglecting to diligently find the correct pills or dosages to accommodate the patients' needs. Yet whether successful or not (very often not) in treating the problems, statistics show that the use of anti-depressants has tripled in the past decade.

What lasting good is being served, where the bottom line is about human beings who's minds and emotions are in shambles!??? Even animals are treated better, with respect to the illness, in our country than most of these people. Only the wealthy ones stand a better chance in more prominent facilities and follow-up care, however the majority of them **do not** have the means for proper treatment. As a result they are reduced to failure after failure (already stockpiled in the psyche) with the meager alternatives, acting out everyone's low expectations including their own. The whole gamut of these unsavory conditions is like a breeding ground for criminal behavior and/or the entrapment and sustaining power of the welfare system. Apparently we are willing to provide **everything except** their foremost need of restoring genuine human dignity, out of the failure to look deep enough into the problems to recognize what is mandatory to accomplish this goal?

What are some of the common threads that tie these misguided souls together? From the onset, as a rule they appear to be more sensitive, even intelligent or creative than the average person. They see, hear, and feel what others miss—with minds like magnets though unable to process correctly all the negativity that permeates society. They can't seem to settle for being ordinary, because somehow they know they are not. They often do not function well in our escalating high-speed, high-tech way of life. It tends to leave them with a cold sense of emptiness. Many possess what poets and artists of all kinds are made of, yet without sincere recognition and guidance, their sensitivity prevents the expression of these valued talents. In a nutshell, it has been said that *"depression is simply unfulfilled desire of the soul"*. Consequently, without this satisfaction, they fall prey to the power of peers and others who drive them into small labeled boxes. They feel stifled. Social acceptance becomes painfully unmanageable. They drop out of the circle, whether quietly or defiantly. They are caught in the Net—food for the predators. No one sees.? No one cares.? And they are on their way—to death, disaster or both...

Another oversimplification of the problem is that there appears to be 2 main categories—those who strike outwardly at others, and those who turn anger inwardly at themselves. Some do not seem to be capable of enduring the pain of depression (or its counterparts) without, at some point, acting out the aggression to the extremes of murder or suicide. Perhaps whether or not they have the inner strength to control their behavior to such drastic ends, depends largely on the values with which they were raised although even there, are many exceptions. While the majority afflicted by these disorders are not considered to be endangering the lives of themselves or others, most of them will spend their whole lifetimes in misery and spreading misery to the people surrounding them. In any case, it is a bleak picture, an epidemic spiraling out of control, having an increasing demoralization on the entire civilized world.

Due to the hidden nature of these disorders, there remains an imminent need for 'scouts' in many corners of society, most importantly in **every** school, who have the training and intuitive ability to recognize the messages that are being exchanged **before** the bitter outcomes. That major issue, to which proper attention is NOT paid, is the **cruelty of youth**, especially toward those who are different or more sensitive, although it is a behavior not only confined to children. It's like a vicious sub-culture that moves about for the sole purpose of exercising destructive power over others to empower themselves. While this enigma is most notable within school surroundings, it is also prevalent in the workplace, and numerous social circles, even religious ones. The pressure is to be forced into "flock" mentality, as opposed to being accepted for personal ideas and values. Because it is often so subtly imposed, it is easily denied and difficult to address, yet none-the-less damaging to a great many receivers. Its as though it has become accepted behavior in our ever-growing hostile environment. The common mind game (even among adults) is to pretend it doesn't exist. In any case, the thrust of that pain is at the heart of <u>every tragic person's story</u>.

The most constant news items are the violent, senseless crimes committed somewhere and everywhere. The prevailing reactions are to get wrapped up in vengeance, or fear that it could have been us, our child, our town… while only few stop to think of the cause. All criminal actions—suicide, murder, rape, child- abduction, domestic violence, hate crimes, on and on, even terrorism, are absolutely rooted in **mental illness**, whether drug or alcohol related or not. The perpetrators are clearly the bold examples of this many-sided disease that has gone untreated, which otherwise could have prevented their grisly actions. The painful truth is that every criminal behind bars or running loose, along with every inmate of our mental institutions did not get to that pathetic stage alone, or overnight. They had a lot of help and time getting there. People somewhere (few or many) aided in bringing them down. And others brought **those** people down…. While the resolve to stop this fateful repetition has been nowhere in place. In one sense our whole country shares the guilt of these crimes, whether out of ignorance or other illusions, by relegating **mental illness** so low on the agenda of **vital issues**.

We pretend to recognize the problems, but the efforts are little more than lip service in light of the overwhelming outcry. Punishment is the best we've had to offer, yet in a way like gasoline to an already raging fire. Where are the real answers in throwing them behind bars or putting them to death, when the numbers are growing faster than we dare to acknowledge? Even if we could scoop them **all** up to be left under lock and key, they will be followed by multitudes at the going rate. For example, look what goes on in our schools—things that were unheard of, even one generation ago. What will **these** kids grow up to be, coming from their culture so filled with empty noise and godless passions? How many more brutalities will it take, by the hands of our own sick fellow citizens alone, before we say with conviction that "enough is enough"? This is the fear side of the equation. Moreover, the fears are justified, not imagined. But if fear can be a motivator for change, then let it serve its rightful purpose and move us into action.

We could do well with a complete overhaul in the perception of 'lost souls'. They are the measuring stick of our priorities (or error therein). The ones who, without cognizance, are leading us to the missing link—**answers that come from wisdom instead of intellect.** If Jesus saw the outcasts of society in the more promising place insofar as being the least resistant to change, thus where He most often demonstrated His greatest compassion, then He must be asking us (who claim to be His followers) to likewise take a closer look. What did He mean by saying, *"Many who are last will be first, and the first last."*? Only the "lost" can know the need to be found, or the "sick" the need of a physician. Perhaps they are in a sense, light bearers to the darkness of their accusers.

We did not learn from Jesus that we were doomed by the forces of evil, but that the power of good was the greater. What then, is it **easier** to sit back and allow evil to flourish? Accept the tragic ironies of ancient philosophies as our destiny as though we have no choice? Or trust that human improvement will somehow inadvertently happen in another lifetime? When it appears to be getting worse? **Today** is the life we know we can count on! And **now** is the time to *"change the things we can"*!—and there are many such things. It seems to be, at that defining point of Grace, where we stumble the most and lose sight of the enormous possibilities/opportunities in our earthly conquests of good over evil.

CHAPTER III

It's strange when you think of it. We wouldn't expect someone with a broken leg to run in a race. Instead the leg would be set promptly by a qualified doctor and given the necessary time to heal. Or victims of cancer and other **physical** diseases are treated by experts with all the latest technology. And support is everywhere. We are also critical, more likely appalled, at religious beliefs that determine to withhold medical attention from those with serious **bodily** needs and illnesses.

Why then is it so difficult to understand the fundamental requirements of healing the obvious wounds in mind and spirit, which are even much more in need of protection from the 'germs of environment' until they are well again? **What is it that keeps us in the dark?** Do we really believe these diseases are incurable? Are we somehow threatened by images of our own secrets if we acknowledge the urgency? Are we afraid of infringing on people's "rights" to live as they please, even when they are not capable of making choices other than destructive ones? Or do we think of addictions and emotional problems of all kinds as moral weakness that deserves punishment—shameful and unworthy of deliberate attention? Even if no crime has yet been committed? If so, then what about all the physical illnesses, caused by the moral weakness of neglect or indulgence, which are readily treated with care and without reservation every day? And what causes more physical deterioration than problems that exist in the mind and emotions? However this in itself is another subject. Aside from that, certainly it would only make good sense to **thoroughly** treat a disease with a risk for crime, against self or others, **before** it happens. Or at least, happens again. To think we can lay claim to giving them a chance by allowing 'a little bit' of help to these prototypes, is as absurd as surgeons who would leave half the cancer in their patients! We should know by now that second rate health care or none at all is much more costly than first rate.??? Undoubtedly when it comes to mental/emotional disorders this is even more so the case. Only the **very best** attention and treatment can produce successful results. As the laws of healing the body take proper time and precautions—so do the laws of healing the mind and spirit.

Sometimes it seems that today's society is floundering in a sea of confusion over everyone's "rights" and "freedoms" that blurs the distinction between inherent right and wrong. There are so many noisy, busy, contradictions that drown out the healthy principles of living life, in which the vast majority have become caught up at some level. Glaring examples are the ever-widening fascinations with the bizarre—exploitation and perversion of sex; graphic themes of horror and violence; repulsive language and behaviors… Rated: For Adults Only, leading kids to believe it's the acceptable prize and conduct on becoming an adult. Why are so many people drawn to entertain the dark side of life, as it plays to an appetite demanding more and worse? And where is the end to worse? In turn, what effect does this "bottom feasting" have on sensitive people, except to often drive them over the edge in all kinds of psychotic manifestations? And so called "normal" people for that matter, if not to desensitize the conscience until it no longer hears what it needs to hear? Perpetually growing more callous and inhumane? <u>If we are to embrace freedom in its entirety, then we must also be prepared to deal responsibly with its pitfalls!</u>

We grapple with who and what is to blame for all the social ills. Is it Parents? Divorce? Schools? Teachers? Churches? Communities? Peer Pressure? Drugs & Alcohol? Television? Movies? Music? Video Games? The Internet? No doubt all of the above and much more are contributors, but ultimately **what good is blame?**

Obviously we can't change all the causes that the majority defends as freedom, and at least <u>appears</u>, able to survive. **But we can change** what we do about those who have lost their way in the maize of infinite causes. Whatever the cause, and in spite of the cause, **it is the cure that should be capturing our attention**. When we can get past the barriers of—Who and What is to blame? Who **deserves** help and how much? What's it gonna cost and Who's gonna pay for it? We're on our way. A shift in focus would indeed be half the battle won.

First of all, it is not a matter of **deserving**, but one of **Grace**, not measured by such terms. Too much time has been wasted, stuck in the misleading rut of shortsightedness toward this growing monumental problem. Single-handedly we cannot help these lost souls no matter now much we care, for the power of the sickness is too great to withstand. Those who suffer from these cruel disorders **need a place**, within our social structure, that is **full of Amazing Grace**—intentionally designed to provide real and lasting recovery. In turn their recovery will eliminate the pain they cause to others. Some will not find it in their hearts to care enough for the 'abusers' to want to give them anything but punishment. Yet conceivably even they, may care enough for the innocent victims of all the hellish drama, or stop to consider that none could become greater healers of others, than those (truly recovered) who once walked in the same shoes.

Secondly, Money is **not** the deciding issue. No reason for red flags or deadlock, because <u>God owns everything</u>! Wherever the resources to begin this effort would come from, the supply is out there (in many forms and coffers) waiting for worthy causes. Beyond that, the inevitable payoff would by far outweigh the cost, and the boundless price we have paid, and still pay.

CHAPTER IV

Albert Einstein once said, *"The consciousness that created the problem cannot be the same consciousness that solves it..."* While this is a spiritual problem, in some ways it need not be approached any differently than any other problem. However, because the components to the solution can only be recognized by the heart, the reasoning must then come from the higher senses. Challenging as it may appear, this creation could render the greatest (long-term, on-going) investment America has ever known, the discovery of a new frontier in the 21st Century. What bigger, better business could we consider? It would *"do us proud"* to embark upon a venture that truly honors the recovery of lost souls.

Perhaps even the key to 'peace on earth' lies within this realm. Although the question may then be, what do we really want more—Peace or Freedom? Each side carries its own price. Yet it seems there should be room for both, that one need not interfere with the other, but rather accommodate the opponent. After all, peace in the hearts of troubled people is simply another choice in the dimension of freedom. A choice that could prevent the uprisings against their falsely perceived enemies. In any case, Peace can only be for those who sincerely want it but have not thus far had a **real opportunity** to experience it. On the other hand, once the opportunity exists for all, who then could predict the number? How many do not seek help because they know of nothing out there, within their means, that is powerful enough to heal their sickness, whether by personal experience or that of others? Although this particular concept of Peace will never appeal to everyone, mainly because complete accountability is at its core, a price many are unwilling to pay. But that too is Freedom's choice. So let it be...

In a television interview many years ago, a renown classical musician and advocate for peace, spoke of Peace as a Middle Road in words to this effect: *"The reason for its difficulty is that we are still over-ruled by extremes. Fanaticism, Liberalism, Materialism, Capitalism, Fundamentalism, Barbarism, so on and so forth.* <u>*Man is not designed to live by extremes*</u>*. However for the Middle to dominate, it must be **stronger than** the SUM of ALL THE EXTREMES—leaving no room for indifference".*

To say God is the answer to all human problems, many believe to be true. Yet to most hopeless people this is much too vague. It is **hands-on** guidance in the finest sense that they need in order to fully recover. We can hardly leave up to God what He has left up to us, and expect miracles to happen. **WE are His miracle workers!** He cannot change this man-made chaos without an incredible man-made transformation of the present-day solutions! whose building blocks must be:

Authentic and Inspired people,
A Place and a Plan of Action,
And Unlimited Resources to empower the Plan into existence.

Wouldn't it be refreshing to see America engaged in a Royal Housecleaning when it comes to the hopeless people, the "burdens (even threats) to society", whose lots we are afraid to acknowledge? The young, the old, the middle-aged. The obvious and the least suspected. Imagine if we were to launch places of healing that surpassed anything ever before dreamed possible! Beyond the barriers of politics and bureaucracy. Beyond the confinements of wealth and class lines. Beyond the disputes of 'left' and 'right' to a common purpose. Beyond the ignorance of discrimination **on all fronts**. Beyond the benevolence of organizations and individuals who strive, even sincerely, to chip away at the problems but are vastly outnumbered or unafforded. Beyond the dogmas of religion, the unending roster of creeds, where technicalities repeatedly breed argument and mistrust (and many with good reason). If there is but one God, why so many versions of Him? Get Him out of the boxes!!! And focus on His Foremost Desire—Genuine Attention to the burning needs of His children all around us! Little by little, heed the outcry! Pull them in from the streets, the schools, the highways and byways, the nursing homes, wherever their living hells exist, with the same single-minded rallying spirit to aid and rebuild the ruins of tornado, flood, earthquake, or war!

A poem entitled "***LOVE***" by an unknown author reads as follows:

> *"There is no difficulty that enough love will not con*
> *quer,*
> *No disease that enough love will not heal,*
> *No door that enough love will not open,*
> *No gulf that enough love will not bridge,*
> *No wall that enough love will not throw down,*
> *No sin that enough love will not redeem.*
> *It makes no difference how deeply seated may be the*
> *trouble,*
> *How hopeless the outlook,*
> *How muddled the tangle ,*

How great the mistake.
*A <u>**SUFFICIENT REALIZATION**</u> of LOVE will dissolve it all.*
*If only you could LOVE <u>**ENOUGH**</u>,*
You would be the happiest and most powerful beings in the world."

Imagine what even a handful of able, inspired people, committed to that level of belief, could do to set the stage for the incredible overture! Wouldn't it be heartening to see as much enthusiasm over curing mind and spirit disease as there is over physical disease? Particularly since **only the body's days are numbered?**

It often seems as though *LOVE* is a four-letter word that is thrown around more carelessly than any other expression today, until it has lost its cutting edge. Yet an interesting fact remains that most people at least appear to understand that somewhere within the same commonly devalued word *LOVE*, lies enough power to change the course of the whole human race if it were ever to be set on fire and turned loose. It's a message that has been heralded for centuries but never as clearly expressed or felt in unison than at the enchanting Christmas Season. An unmistakable magic fills the air as though the world stops on its path for a moment while heaven and earth embrace the entire human family to summon their finest senses…

LOVE in its highest form is the divine substance we have access to, and the only hope of healing our social illnesses. However by its very nature it must be structured and channeled in right directions that go straight to the heart of the problem, in order to accomplish its mission. Most people are too busy living life, consumed by work and play, to even begin to recognize the enormity of this power. The tendency is that Love has become confined to families, close friends, falling in love…, even God in an exclusive sort of way. All of this has by some measure, diverted the incredible energy of its intention to heal beyond these circles. Only in times of great trial and hardship, if then, are we able to fathom the capabilities of Love, the purity of its God-like qualities, and from Whence it comes to us.

CHAPTER V

It's impossible to fully explain the force of reasoning behind the vision called A Manor of Eden, other than to say that it evolved from the pain of feeling, hearing, and seeing the pain in others, beginning with those closest to me. I had also served my own term in the bottomless pit of depression at one time—the indescribable suffering, outweighed by none other. Although the greatest torment in that state of mind was to find nothing or no one to help ease the pain. Only an instinctive guidance from within would finally bring me to the other side. It is one thing to personally experience this agony, far another when it touches your child.

Eating disorders still remain the most severely underrated of all addictions, therefore they run rampant in society. Though powerful in grip and dangerous in effect, they are the easiest to disguise. What could go more unnoticed in a world so enamored by FOOD? The cross-over between bulimia and anorexia is the addiction I have witnessed most closely. It is **real!** and it is **ruthless!** Plus it often invites other addictions to subdue its control. My youngest daughter Kelly was 14 when the bulimic symptoms began, after moving from a small mid-western town to Seattle. Before this unexpected invasion she was the kind of lovely, endearing child any parent would wish for—so full of vitality and talent, as were all 3 of the children. The outset was at a time when I believed we had all made it through the rain, the sleet, the snow... However it would prove to be the greatest humbling experience of my life.

I was a single parent (since they were very young) with no financial or moral support from their father, and totally unprepared for the road ahead. Besides recognizing the need to conquer my own erroneous zones, I set out to prove that loving my children, trying hard, encouraging the 'right' things, raising them in the church, and a lot of prayers, would save them from the grim statistics. Yet contrary to even the best efforts and intentions, the most overwhelming helplessness was that there were always far too many factors beyond my reach as a parent.

There are no words to describe the horrors of Kelly's escalating multiple addictions, depraved lifestyles, abusive relationships and behavior, and numerous suicide attempts, that proceeded over the following (now) twenty years since her struggle began. The black cloud hung relentlessly overhead, leaving its mark on every family member. High hopes were dashed throughout all the inpatient (presently 11) and outpatient treatments, the changing myriad of anti-depressants, 12-step programs, counseling, religious experiences, support and prayers of friends, relatives and well-meaning people... Periodically (and still) out of desperation Kelly would come home and I could not find it in my heart to turn my back on her, as though part of my purpose was to keep her alive. Comfort was often simply knowing she was safe. It was not uncommon in her precarious situations elsewhere to keep vigilance until dawn praying (if only) for her protection. Certainly somewhere within the miracle of Amazing Grace lies the reason Kelly is still alive today. And I **Thank God** for that!

For the most part, all 'normalcy' to life progressively ended during those years. Other than the ability to perform my duties at work and the everyday tasks of living, staying in touch with a dwindling number of friends and family members, I became consumed with a passion to understand the nature of Kelly's disease, the similarity of others, and all that empowered them. Everything else fell to the bottom of the priority list... It was an endless parade of reading, observing, listening to experts, listening to reason and experience, listening to all kinds of people including the victims, and last but not least—listening and talking to God. It was a feeling that **would not** rest, year after year, both agonizing and rewarding. Somewhere amidst the insatiable, often grueling emotions, was like a force pushing me onward, yet where it would lead was mainly unclear. It was also a lonely road. Attempts at discussion had many times proven futile by criticism or ideas that went unheard. It appears to be a subject most people choose to avoid, certainly at a level with real disclosure. It became less painful not to be reminded that my heartfelt interests were not commonly shared. The cocoon slowly spun itself around me, all the while believing that someday the time would come to venture out on the wings of expression, if only in the pages of a book. Nevertheless, had it not seemed right to pursue this path, initially driven by the love I held for Kelly, and all my children for that matter, I would not have experienced the manifestation of A Manor of Eden.

It happened during one of Kelly's most critical interludes, at a time when I was first able to face the heart-wrenching reality that she was bound for death, with no answers left in sight. I was home alone one evening, feeling overpowered with fear. However hard to explain, suddenly an aura of Grace began to fill the room and I became astounded by what I saw. The most intense, enlightening picture proceeded to surround me—clear as glass, and one that could never be erased. But it wasn't just about Kelly, it was about everyone who suffered from these ravaging diseases. It was a place that held the answers to every mental and emotional problem, **right here on earth**. The whole phenomenon was amazing, yet incredibly basic and full of detail. For every question that raced through my mind, there was an answer and extension to the picture. There were provisions and solutions for any problem that could arise, such as the importance of healing the family members as well. Nothing was left out. Truly it was the most intimate, humbling experience I could have imagined, to the extent that it was impossible to share it meaningfully with any other known human being.

It is without reason to believe that I witnessed any of this for simply a personal escape from "reality" on a dark day. Considering the innumerable dark days over many years prior, **never** had there been such an encounter. Yet since then, I've felt deep inside that I was obliged to tell the story that has changed my perspectives toward these dreadful diseases **forever**. Knowing that even if the sole outcome would be to sing **my "heart song"** while on this earth, it was still a duty impossible to avoid. The greatest difficulty by far, has been the task of putting the picture into words for the clarity of others, especially the unmistakable healing Spirit (the perfect mix of strength, tenderness, peace, trust, order...) that lingered everywhere, within the place, within the people—the very essence of what made it so outstanding. And beyond that, how does one convey the countless technicalities which were of equal significance, without diminishing the powerful nature of it all? The formidable mountain, yet in the end did not defeat the purpose.

The vision has been written in present tense (as seen in the mind's eye) with its great potential for development over time. To understand the enormous possibilities of such a Place, is simply a matter or raising one's level of consciousness. Why is it this seems to be so much easier in the challenges of Scientific endeavors? We should know by now that **'ordinary'**, conservative thinking cannot fix these kinds of problems, even though the answers are neither complex nor illogical. Although certainly not everyone is meant to concern themselves with issues of this sort, but for **those who are**—a new and uncommon wisdom **must come into view.** Why not rise to a higher level of ideals when there is so much at stake? What is there to lose? Another question is, where do people and leaders in churches, temples, mosques...really stand on these undeniably spiritual problems? While such associations are not equipped to handle all the profound, individual needs, what would be their support of a common purpose? To appeal to the consciousness of Christians alone, what did Jesus ever do that was **'ordinary'** in the face of human impossibilities? He raised people from the dead; made the blind see and the lame walk; cast out demons; fed 5000 people with 5 loaves and 2 fish;... and said **"Follow Me"**. Then later on before He left— "Even greater things than these can you do when I'm gone, if you will just **believe"**... Wouldn't He see all the mental and emotional illnesses of today just as (if not more) worthy of healing as those of the body? Has our faith become so small, strayed so far from our Leaders intentions that we don't hear the outcry? Never has a more compelling illustration of LOVE been portrayed than *The PASSION of the Christ.* After such a jolt to the senses, how can we **not** believe that the same Power is still available, waiting for human visionaries to take action against the most troublesome (yet concealed and denied) of all pain?

What you are about to read would not be greater than any **one** of Jesus' miracles—only greater in number and proportion. Although words seem inadequate, the following pages contain my best attempt to describe the vision as operating in its full-grown capacity...

PART II

A MANOR OF EDEN

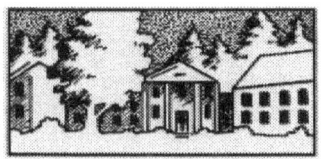

A MANOR OF EDEN is the given name to an extraordinary vision of healing the diseases of mind and spirit. While these afflictions are commonly thought of in many isolated terms, they are treated as various forms of One Problem—namely Misguided People who have lost their way. The remarkable success rate is due to the necessary elements of recovery being carried out to the fullest measure—anchored in many beliefs such as:

    All people are born with equal value—
        Every life is worth saving.
        Every person, when restored, has untold potential for good.
        No human being is a hopeless case.

    God's intention for all of His children, <u>with no exception</u>, far exceeds the heart of the soundest earthly parent—
        Wholeness,
        True Happiness,
        A life contributing to the good of humanity.

    The mind and spirit (just as the body), are designed by the Creator to heal themselves—
        When all negative stimuli is removed,
        Thoroughly replaced with positive experience,
        And allowed to crystallize for an <u>essential</u> length of time.

The only way to produce total wellness is to treat all separate components of the whole, simultaneously, as opposed to dissecting the person and giving more attention to one than the other two—
Body,
Mind,
Spirit.

When personal value is truly reclaimed, the soul emerges with freedom to—
Touch the finger of God (again),
Dream great dreams,
And release the power to make them come true.

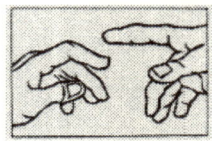

CERTAIN HIGH-LIGHTS AND DETAILS AS SEEN IN THE VISION ARE RECORDED HERE, ALTHOUGH MANY TECHNICALITIES ARE NOT INCLUDED AT THIS TIME.

To begin with—A simple "back to basics" routine is elevated to a high level of excellence. The program is based on sound and proven techniques of experts in every area and implemented in an environment that breeds wellness to all the senses. The process is comparable to a condensed version of growing up within the guidance of a healthy, secure, and loving home, by paying full attention to the needs which have not been met. The traditional Twelve Steps are also embraced in the program. The credentials of every worker, professional and otherwise, are of the finest quality and intentions of the heart, affirming in action that **no half measures will suffice.** They are sincerely dedicated to the entire backbone of the institution which is THE HIGHER THE IDEALS, THE GREATER THE RESULTS.

The program is divided into four distinct categories:

Stage 1—Dealing in depth with the past

Stage 2—Recovering the wisdom and values of the inner-child

Stage 3—Developing knowledge for healthy living

Stage 4—Formal education, job training, and job placement

More details on each of these phases are noted later in the description.

Not until Stage 4 does the program become co-educational. Prior to this, men and women remain completely separated. All workers and staff members are required to go through Stages 1—3, if for no other reason than to become familiar with the exact treatment of the patients, although the experience in itself would give benefit to anyone.

No one is turned away or treated any differently for lack of resources upon entering this facility. The only admission requirement is a sincere desire to positively change one's life within the standards of A Manor of Eden. When the program is successfully completed and the graduates are engaged in gainful employment, a re-payment plan is set up based on the cost of their particular length of treatment. However this provision does not apply to those who **do** have the means with which to pay. Also in situations concerning child care as a deciding point of **not** making the commitment, arrangements are available to provide 24-hour, nurturing, quality care of the children **including those with special needs** (under such necessary circumstances) while the parent is isolated from the family in order to fully concentrate on their own personal recovery.

The important factor of diet is introduced in the beginning and continues its significance throughout the program. It is portrayed with an attitude that eating is simply a routine necessity to nourish and refuel the body. However mealtime involves a happy atmosphere knowing that only wholesome food is aiding to produce wellness in body, mind and spirit, therefore a very essential part of recovery. Education on nutritional value is to produce a factual understanding of this connection. The goal is first to eliminate all physical causes of mental and emotional conflict, and the results over a reasonable period of time are often phenomenal.

For the first few days the diet is composed primarily of freshly extracted fruit and vegetable juices for the ease of digestion, detoxification, and hastening of the recovery process. After that, the meals are carefully selected from various sources, masters in the field of nutrition, including that of Dr. Paul Bragg, grandfather of physical fitness, and others with more recent discoveries. Special attention is given to balancing food combinations, drinking pure spring water in adequate amounts, and the intake of natural, plant-source, vitamin and mineral supplements. In the advanced Stages 3 and 4, periodic (short-term) fasting is introduced to most patients and monitored by professionals. This training also defines the importance of exercise, along with fresh air and sunshine. Physical exercise activities vary with the different stages—in Stage 1 mainly walking, jogging, Yoga... Later on they include swimming, team sports, various types of dance... and always remain an essential part of the program.

Considerable emphasis is placed on development of the **individual**, based on the premise that relationships cannot be successful, especially those of intimacy, until we are first complete within ourselves. Therefore no communication with outside friends or family members is permitted for 90 days and is then carefully evaluated by the counselors. It is highly recommended that the spouse or intimate partner goes through the program as well, in order to maintain a new healthy relationship and to ensure the on-going stability of the patient.

Past traditions and values are connected to the present,

believing that the lack of present built on past, constitutes a lost society. National and religious holidays are celebrated in rich and heartfelt fashion. Sounds and visuals are given special regard—well-rounded yet absent of negative overtones concerning music, entertainment, pictures, books, movies...Soft, tranquil music plays throughout the buildings, including the patients' rooms.

If it appears that the 'strong' have a choice to manage life without sound discipline and a personal relationship with God, it is for certain the 'weak' are hopeless in their absence. However it is of utmost importance that the perception of God be seen in His truly magnificent nature—the loving, caring Father of all who seek to know Him. Although the foundation of the institution is framed by the Christian faith, the patients <u>are not</u> taught religious doctrine. But they <u>are</u> taught the fundamentals of living life as honorable human beings with real value, based on the wisdom of solid, time-tested principles from the Bible and other holy books. The intention is to break down the dividing barriers and embrace all trustworthy features that many religions have in common.

One hour a day is set aside for group worship and instruction. This is officiated by a clergyman who instills the significance of building strong character, relating everything that is taught in the program from a spiritual perspective. It is very positively approached, as well as grounded for the benefit of all. This takes place in the chapel, a quaint and charming place, enhanced with many wonderful attributes: a bell tower, stained glass windows, pipe organ, candelabras, a large wooden cross, a statute of a Shepherd and sheep, the American Flag, a life-size Eagle sculpture, a replica of stone tablets with *The Ten Commandments*, several richly framed verses including *The Lord's Prayer*, *The 23rd Psalm*, *The Golden Rule*, the poem *Love*…. Chimes ring out across the grounds every morning before chapel and other times throughout the day with a diversity of patriotic melodies, traditional songs and hymns such as *A Mighty Fortress Is Our God, America the Beautiful, Battle Hymn of the Republic*… The glow of peace, honor and clarity fills the air and hearts of all within this captive range. Upon arising and before bedtime there is also time reserved for private prayer and meditation. All of these spiritual experiences are highly nurturing to the patients and play the most significant role in their recovery.

The essence of A Manor of Eden is the unique ability of its leaders to administer the entire treatment program with remarkable skill and insight. Their undivided attention to the needs of each person contributes to the healing spirit that abides everywhere. The presentation is straight-forward, not designed to stir up the emotions with disorderly, unrealistic persuasions, but one that stabilizes, strengthens and gives clear understanding to the value of emotions. Although well compensated for their work, no one in the organization is guided by the entrapments of fame or fortune. In this place such motives are simply non-existent. Instead the leaders are guided by the wisdom of humility and honor in their chosen services.

The following is a summarization of the recovery process, beginning with Stage l.

Normally the length of this phase is 28 days. However, if at the end of any stage, particularly the first, there is need for a patient to continue on for a longer period of time, this would happen on the recommendations of the assigned professionals who carefully monitor the progress of each individual.

Stage 1, After Admission:

- Detoxification from drugs or alcohol for 72 hours (if necessary) under doctor and nurse's surveillance.
- Complete physical examination by a medical doctor.
- Written psychological testing administered and evaluated by a psychiatrist followed by an introductory 2 hour session.
- Medications are available if necessary, with a goal to eliminate whenever possible.
- Assessment with an attorney, who acts as a mediator on any pending legal, financial, or employment leave-of-absence issues which the patient might have.
- Assignment of a personal Guardian. The Guardians are carefully matched and selected from the graduates of Stage 3, who in addition have completed an intensive training course. They are the main companion and guide to their entrusted patients throughout the program, particularly in Stage 1.
- The patients are assigned to their own private rooms and given a colorful array of red, white & blue uni-

forms, appropriated for various activities. The purpose of uniforms is to symbolize equality and accentuate likeness rather than difference in human problems and their recovery.
- Orientation involves a series of lectures and films describing in detail the plan, rules, and purpose of the institution. General expected behavior is clearly defined, along with disciplinary action in terms of manners & grooming; no criticism of others or 'clannish clicks' are acceptable, nor use of foul language anywhere outside the private counseling offices.
- Daily 1 hour, one-on-one private counseling with a fully certified therapist.
- Daily 2 hour small-group sessions (6—8 patients) under the supervision of well qualified leaders. The groups are organized according to the type of addiction and/or problem level. Cigarette smoking cessation is also incorporated into these sessions and eliminated by the end of 28 days or before.
- Positive group lectures conducted by guest speakers or staff professionals on dealing with past negative behaviors.
- Weekly 1 hour private sessions with the psychiatrist who has all the updated information on the patient.
- At the end of 28 days—2nd complete physical examination and 2nd written psychological test for re-evaluation.

Stage 2—

The purpose of this 28-day period is to bring the patients back to the reality of childhood experience for re-connection with that vital part of themselves. Each one is required to bring with them 3 favorite pictures (if available), at age levels 1-2 years, 4-5 years, and 8-9 years which are mounted in clear view in their rooms. Basically the patients learn to see this inner-child as the wonder-filled place where there are no 'lids' nor contamination to undermine the truth about who they are. The place where 'realness' abides, the connection to God—conscience, faith, imagination, sensitivity, creativity… Jesus said, *"Except you become as little children, you cannot see the kingdom of God"*—the soul/the true self. It is within these kinds of concepts that the patients develop a sound foundation, a genuine sense of personal value on which to rebuild their lives. **And above all, they learn how to 'Keep it Simple'…**

Activities include:
- Enjoying a small 'McDonald's Farm' along with caring for the animals. Bird-watching and feeding…
- Taking care of the vegetable and flower gardens— weeding, watering, and learning the fundamentals about plants.
- Developing the consciousness of the intended relationship between all of nature and human beings.
- Basic cooking lessons and helping in the kitchen with meal preparation.
- 2 days a week, 1 hour of one-on-one private counseling sessions.
- 3 days a week, 2 hour small-group counseling, geared to recognizing the 'child' strengths and values as an

adult.
- Two 1-hour sessions with the psychiatrist—end of 2 weeks and end of 4 weeks.

Stage 3 —

This 28-day period is primarily to build upon the principles learned in Stages 1 and 2. Here the patients are given additional tools with which to live life as honorable adults. Much of this is in the form of positive group lectures on all kinds of topics and recovery issues, often conducted by professional guest speakers. These subjects are also discussed at length each day within the small-group sessions.

It is in Stage 3 that a real understanding of the program melds together. Clearly, fitness of the whole person is the only way for lasting change to occur. Out of that change comes the healthy desire to earn an honest wage in a job that is satisfying to each individual. One of the main goals is that every graduate will never again (if before) find it necessary to be a statistic on the welfare rolls.

Activities include:
- Once a week, 1 hour of one-on-one private counseling sessions
- Daily 2 hour small-group counseling and discussions.
- Assigned reading and written reports
- Movies (entertainment & educational)
- Extended exercise and sports activities
- Two 1-hour sessions with the psychiatrist—end of 2 weeks and end of 4 weeks.
- End of Stage 3—3rd written psychological test and re-evaluation.

Additional activities on weekends for all recovery stages:

- Appreciation of Music, Literature and Arts classes
- Professional music concerts or other performances
- Inspirational Songfests around a campfire or fireplace (depending on weather or season) often conducted by guest artists.

Engaging the Family:

After graduation from Stage 3, a 14—21 day (depending on need) family involvement program takes place, in which spouses, close friends, and family members are clearly educated on the entire treatment plan and purpose. They attend chapel, meals and certain other activities with their respective patients, including daily private and group family counseling sessions. Wherever there are obvious problems within the unit, particularly with the spouse, the counselor strongly recommends the need for these family members to go through the full treatment program themselves. Housing is available to these individuals during the time of intervention, outside the facility grounds. They are also encouraged to become involved in the support groups established throughout the country, all hosted by professionals within the organization. These groups are designed to provide an unbroken connection and after-care for the graduates of the treatment program as well as a great benefit to the entire family.

10-day Training for Becoming Guardians—

This class is for all patients that have successfully completed Stage 3. It is taught by professionals, who at the end of the course submit an evaluation of each student to the psychiatrist, who in turn assigns the Guardians to new patients.

Stage 4—

This part of the program is optional and depends solely on the individual's educational background, personal circumstances, or desire to make changes in their present line of work. If they are without a job and choose to leave when Guardianship is completed, they are referred to the placement service within the organization that is registered with employment agencies throughout the country. These agencies hold special regard for A Manor of Eden and highly recommend the graduates of this program. The policy is that **no one** will leave the institution without full-time employment awaiting them if they are financially responsible for themselves or their families.

For those who choose to stay, this is a highly accredited educational system, ranging from high school through college, including training in various occupational trades. The instructors are all excellent quality professionals. The positive personal concern for every student continues on in the exact manner as the treatment program. Class advisors and counselors are always available. The students are tested for vocational interests and abilities and given an abundance of career counseling. They are also placed in part-time jobs within the organization, coordinated by their particular schedules, which allows them to earn room & board and tuition while attending school.

Within this framework the cycle perpetuates its unending goal—to heal the spirits of the afflicted so they may become instruments of healing others and rebuild their own lives with real purpose and meaning. Given time, the contributions of these restored individuals will filter back into society a much needed set of values.

A Manor of Eden will evolve into a self-sustaining entity to include diversified industries and professions, first of all to serve the various needs of the institution and secondly for the development of reproductions in other locations. A matter of primary importance is to ensure that the number of patients in each facility is always kept at an effective personal level. The end result will offer a growing number of jobs to those who need or choose them at the completion of their respective programs, in addition to the jobs held by students during their education. In a practical sense, certainly it would also by definition *"boost the American economy"* in the process. However the foremost intention is that each person with their own unique abilities, will have the guidance and opportunity to live useful, productive lives, and make dreams come true. This is a timeless institution for everyone who enters its bounds—to freely remain within the structure of employment; resume a rightful place in society outside its gates; or return and contribute to the infinite objective.

Finally, the goal is to carry this extraordinary vision of recovery, in all ways possible, into prisons and mental institutions, where confinement is mandatory. By virtue of its principles alone, such incredible needs could not be ignored. The firm belief that no human being is hopeless or unworthy of compassionate care, stands entirely on the strength of character and commitment; deep and abiding capacity to Love; and unwavering faith in God, all of which are held by **every member** of the organization. Therein rests the heart and power of the mission…

AN OVERVIEW—AFTER 911

A Manor of Eden is much more than a *"field of dreams"* or a wonderful figment of imagination. Not only is it entirely possible, but it is **destined** to become a whole new industry in itself—a God-inspired industry of restoring people from their hopeless conditions, back to the dignity for which they were born. The concepts of failure and mediocrity will not survive a genuine resolve toward excellence, for the same reason that demons flee when faced with the bold light of Truth.

This simple blueprint of ideas may be likened to *"the 5 loaves and 2 fishes"*. In due time, when authentic visionaries see the greatest challenge in the world today through the eyes of the Creator, they will gladly roll up their sleeves to make miracles happen. By a strategic move from *default to purpose,* A Manor of Eden could be transformed from an aspiring image to a **real *OPERATION of SOUL RECOVERY*.** Accordingly God, with His eminent capacity to Love, would open the floodgates of blessing upon this lofty goal. To all who believe in the American Dream—if there was ever one to set the record straight and lead the way in the 21st Century, this is at least a place to begin. There could be no better way to heal our land, than a willful plan to undermine the infectious roots of evil, set the captives free, and add credible substance to the appeal that truly "***No one* is left behind**". That would be **N**ational **S**ecurity at its best!— for *"we are only as strong as our weakest links"*…

America is like a glass house for all the world to see. **What is it** our enemies see that fuels such **passion** to destroy us? Is it possible that ignoring the blatant need to first clean up our own dingy corners and caves may have something to do with it? The War on Terror should be the signal to include this forsaken element, for it runs hand in hand with the intention. Passion, gone awry, is basically what every 'ism' and addiction is about, be it Drugs, Alcoholism, Satanism, Terrorism or any other 'ism' of deception including those in the names of many religions. Until we can see clearly the connection between mental/emotional disorders & threatening movements, and **all criminal acts of violence** (that are as closely related as life and breath) there can be no such thing as peace—only more violence and the lust for punishment and revenge.

As the great leader we are, why not give the peering world, <u>especially our enemies</u>, a brand new precedent on which to ponder, by the way we handle **soul sickness** within our own shores? How much more desperate (in too many regions) are the needs of **their** children who are constantly falling prey to the fangs of extremism, often carried out to the barbaric end of being used as suicide bombers. Whether or not there is a valid time and place for war is debatable, however the long-term solution to **peace** goes far beyond these ruthless measures. In any event, **now** is a momentous time to **make peace**, (even if it must be amidst the winds of war). But it <u>will not</u> happen **until we <u>make</u> it happen**! As the misguided, angry masses lose hope for the dawning of a new day, we could begin to establish the making of such a day.

If America has failed most at anything, it is that we have turned our backs on the plight of the lost and vulnerable and left them to gravitate toward all kinds of predators.

We cannot take away the false 'fixes' and expect success, without replacing these passions with something even more powerful and obviously for Good. Every citizen of this country should have the right to know that there is a **trusted** Place to go in times of trouble, just as assuredly as knowing where to go in times of physical emergency, whether it be for themselves or a loved one. We will have succeeded when there is such a Place in **every** locality, that is well equipped for the business of taking seriously the healing of all troubled souls.

There could be no price tag comparable to the ones we have paid for decades, with too little thought, but where have they led us? In our arrogance we've been blinded by all kinds of intellectual thinking which lacks compassion—clinical ideas far removed from the problems, monetary shortsightedness, that could only be calculated by 'adult' minds. We leave the real, defining answers to children, who are in many ways wiser and closer to the angels than any grownup. I wonder how many 'older folks' recall a song with the lyrics, *"I will make you fishers of men, if you follow Me..."* which once upon a time we sang so robustly—straight from the heart, as we did many others with equal value. Yet we brush these memories aside, because now they seem to interfere with most everything we have learned to call 'reality', choosing instead to ignore the counsel of scripture that says, *"and a little child shall lead them"*.

No finer classic examples have sought to grace the world with simple truth, than little Mattie Stepanek with his lovely collection of *"Heart Songs"* and visions of peace, who began his writings at the age of two, despite battling an incurable disease; or young Billy Gilman's most heartening rendition of *"My Time on Earth"*. In view of all the senseless unrest, how do we process these timely messages from the mouths of innocence, that shower our hearts with tears of enlightenment, and **EVER** go back to *"business as usual"* again??? Certainly, we could use a huge dose of their wisdom here and now. And frankly all of these insightful children **need our help!** While it may sound so naïve to some, so much like cockeyed optimism, one does not have to know all the nuts and bolts to know they are merely the details that take care of themselves in the big picture. What the world needs more than ever before, is **a whole regiment of cockeyed optimists** who would stand fearless and unyielding against the cynics, for a cause determined to recover **peace** in the hearts of people! Without time limits, and with the will to *"go the distance"*.

Jesus said, *"Blest are the peacemakers...,* and *Blest are those who hunger and thirst for what is right and good, for they shall be satisfied."* He also told us the order of succession, *"Do not be overcome by evil, but overcome evil with good"*. **What** are we waiting for???

Combat against evil, wherever or however it thrives, is to recognize its ability to maneuver, and with that wisdom, fight the good fight with revolutionizing commitment, until these vagrant adversaries crumble, like the walls of Jericho! Although it is not simply people we are at war with, but the distortion in their minds.

Nevertheless we can be certain from the outset that the enemy will at last **be** defeated because the towering Commander will forever stand on the winning side of **J**ustice, **G**oodness, and **T**ruth. Ultimately God is the Leader who beats the drum, that stirs the hearts, that follow the sounds of the perfect dream—**Peace on His Beloved Earth...**

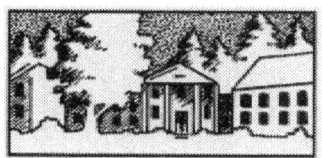

"IF WE BUILD IT, HE WILL COME"....
To help us clean up America! so all the greatness can shine forth brilliantly, like a beacon of hope for other nations as well...

"You are the Salt of the Earth."

"You are the Light of the World."

"What you will do for the least of my brothers, you will do for Me."

"Go therefore to the streets and thoroughfares and invite all you can find, both bad and good, to the marriage feast."

"Those who are well have no need of a physician, but those who are sick."

"And even greater things than these, will you do when I'm gone."

"If you have faith as a grain of mustard seed, you can say to this mountain, 'move', and <u>nothing</u> shall be impossible to you."

Matthew, Mark, Luke, John—

PART III

ABOUT THE AUTHOR

Sheryl Stevens was born and raised in a well regarded midwestern family. She attained a college degree in Business Administration, which led to working primarily in the field of accounting, besides several years of employment in social service positions. Sheryl is the mother of three grown children, along with one grandson. She was formerly a fifteen-year resident of southern California, returned to her hometown in North Dakota for nine years, and since then has resided in Seattle, Washington.

THE LOGIC OF VISIONS

Perhaps there is not nearly as much mystery in visions as some are inclined to think. When 'everyday' reasoning power is broken down, due to extreme circumstances, occasionally it's as though the subconscious dumps itself into the consciousness. If allowed to proceed, all knowledge and experiences regarding the desperate situation, including a wisdom beyond oneself, seem to be called forth at the same time, which brings into focus a very real picture that ordinarily could not be seen. Visions are exclusive to each occurrence—never before nor after to be perceived in that exact light. It also seems clear that they contain messages of hope, **from God**, simply because the barriers between God and humankind have momentarily disappeared. Therefore they are worthy of attention.

The following is a condensed narrative of personal experiences, beginning with a collection of childhood memories written in 1993. A number of these happenings, along with many others, seem now to have greatly influenced A Manor of Eden, both directly and indirectly as part of its unique symmetry.

"ONCE UPON A TIME—

From a long line of hardy Norwegians I came. Adventuresome grandparents on both sides. Migrants from the old country. Homesteaders in Midwestern America. Perhaps the trace of Viking blood was also a boon to my survival, although I suppose one never really knows such things.

It was a perfect little spot on the earth. 140 acres nestled back within the hills, many miles north of a small town in North Dakota, close to the Canadian border. In countless ways it was like a **Garden of Eden**. Heavily wooded with trees and bushes; meadows, wildflowers and berries; green pastures with grazing cattle and horses; miniature fields (as compared to the prairie farms) of waiving grain, alfalfa, sweet clover; a large potato patch; a vegetable garden...

The house sat on top of a hill. Four small rooms downstairs. A tiny kitchen with a wood-burning cook stove; a wash stand and basin in one corner; and a little enamel-topped table in front of the north window that overlooked the front yard and a glimpse of the highway through the trees. Descending from the pantry was a root cellar where an abundance of harvest was carefully stored. A huge bin of potatoes; shelves lined with home-canned jams and jellies, fruits and vegetables. Smoked ham and bacon slabs hung from the ceiling. A large stone jar of home-churned butter stood at the foot of the steep stairway. The upstairs was simply a bare-rafter attic, which my brother and I shared for bedrooms. His was the north end, mine the south, crudely partitioned midway at the chimney.

The log barn was down the hill at the end of a tree-lined path. I loved the feeling, even the smell in the barn, always clean and well kept. Dad had a certain affection for his cattle and other livestock that I never sensed as much elsewhere. They were all meticulously fed, bedded down with straw and cared for. Thereby the animals were gentle, contented-looking creatures. Even in the dead of winter it was a warm and comfortable place to be—with a sort of hush in the air that must have been in another stable one night long ago.

Water was fetched for its appropriate use from the rain barrels in summer, melted snow in winter, or the hard-water well down the hill. Our bathroom was an outhouse, equipped with discarded Sears & Roebuck catalogues. Kerosene lamps and lanterns were our lights, coal and wood our heat. Everything was done in a simple and orderly manner. We were not poor, just average in comparison to others in the neighborhood.

Dad was an honest hard-working farmer. A rather quiet man, at least where I was concerned. His formal education ended in the 8th grade, not unusual in that he was the eldest of seven children when his mother died. Therefore he became the right-hand man to HIS father, who was somewhat of a disagreeable, hard-to-please old chap. Although in spite of his burly character, Grandpa was never very convincing he was a man without heart. I admired him—though usually from a distance. Dad's family was the earthy type. Devoted farmers, early risers, jokers with hearty laughter, relished their tobacco plugs (the men that is), handsome & leathery on the outside, and highly respected folks of the "old" Lutheran faith.

Mom's family, on the other hand, was a more refined, classy sort. Well educated, high spirited, musically inclined, poetic... Their religion was that of an off-shoot of the Lutheran church, very dogmatic and persuasive, by which they had all been thoroughly indoctrinated. My mother was one of seven sisters and a brother. A graceful attractive lady. Raised in Minnesota and later ventured west to the rugged wilds of ND with her sister to teach school, where they eventually married two of the dashing brothers and settled.

Mom continued her teaching career in the surrounding country schools (except for the one I attended) throughout my growing up years. Very dedicated, very much in demand. Sincerity and whole-heartedness was the way she did everything, including the endless hours at the dining room table preparing worksheets for her "school children", correcting papers, marking report cards, all with neat and precise accomplishment. She'd make regular visits to the homes of these children, especially the less fortunate ones, for encouragement reasons. And I would often tag along. She was a wonderful cook and baker, very festive, enthusiastic, sensitive. Everyone loved and respected Mom. I was always proud of her. My mother was **everything** I wanted to be.

My brother was four years older than I. A handsome lad, well-mannered, intelligent. Read books by lamplight until wee hours of the morning. Sang and played the guitar. In all respects the more promising child. Although he tolerated me most of the time, we were like apples and oranges.

I was rather a comic-looking, freckle-faced kid. Straight hair and pigtails. Strong willed, often painfully shy around grownups. A dreamer, an artist at make-believe. Never bored, never lonely. And always drinking in to my ever-so-keen senses, the awesome world around me:

I REMEMBER....

The sound of poplar leaves rustling in the wind. The smell of wild pink roses after a rain. How refreshing they looked with tiny droplets on the petals. Buttermilk clouds against the blue sky, especially at sunrise, or watching a golden sunset streaming through the westward trees. The intriguing splendor of a clear night. The crescent moon. The full moon. The endless stars, like shiny little windows to a magic land...

Dashing through the woods pretending I was a deer, wishing to be as graceful. Catching a baby cottontail and holding it gently in my hands. I loved the smell of puppies' breath, their little pink tongues licking my face. Trailing behind Patty, the obliging cattle dog, as she drove the lazy cows home for milking. A wobbly-legged calf sucking my fingers. Gathering eggs from the nests of sassy hens.

Feeding the little motherless fawn from a baby bottle. Dad found him in the woods one day and carried him home. A tame and sleek beauty he grew to be and lost his spots. Licked the salt blocks and romped with the young cattle like he was one of them.

Picking violets that liked those shady mossy places, or hunting four-leaf clovers. A time when dandelions were still a beautiful bouquet of flowers to brighten the dinner table. Biting off the tasty tips of honey-suckles, or grimacing with a mouth full of gooseberries. Running barefoot in the grass after a thunderstorm. Chasing the mystic colours of a rainbow.

The smell of clean clothes drying in the breeze, or Mom's fresh brown bread just out of the oven. Rushing to the kitchen for a warm jam sandwich. The summertime playhouses in the woods, with stumps for chairs and table-legs, a jug with a cork for running water. Baking mud pies in an oven made of rocks. My dolls were "real people"—they talked, they laughed, they cried, and shared my love of fairy tales.

In winter, the way the frost clung lavishly to the branches, like prisms creating delightful colours as the sun shined. Ice skating on the ponds and meadows. Drawing pictures on frosted window panes. Thick quilts and warm flatirons at the foot of the bed.

On bitter cold days when the snowdrifts were insurmountable by car, riding to school in the horse-drawn cutter. Through the small window I could see Prince and Charm dancing friskily while they awaited our seating. They looked happy with their frosty whiskers, and white smoke billowing from their nostrils, as I sat on a soft bed of hay, cuddled snugly under the heavy felt-lined horsehide blanket. The squeaking sound of the runners gliding across the hard-packed snow, the clippity-clop of the horses feet and jingling harnesses.

I loved the wintertime, and especially at school. Playing in snow-houses carved out of gigantic banks, with endless tunnels and cozy rooms. Building forts to shield snowball fights; darting around the pie in the game of fox & geese; making jolly snowmen; skating on the snow-cleared patch of frozen lake across the road; sliding down hills on sleds or toboggans with woolen scarves wound tightly around our faces.

The country schoolhouse was 2 miles from home, where a single room served all eight grades with an entire group of 10—15 children. The old wooden desks with carved initials on the top. Inkwells and fountain pens. The smell of books and crayons, sticky jars of paste, and peanut butter sandwiches. For the most part I liked school, although I didn't care much to study. I was average.

Whereas I delighted in all the frivolous play at recess, there were other things that felt very comfortable. It was a time when the Golden Rule was branded to every small conscience and still made uncomplicated sense. When the reading of scripture introduced each school day. And the aura of patriotism graced the air, making the faces of Washington and Lincoln come alive as they looked kindly at us from their high posts above the blackboard. I was a proud little American. Reciting the Pledge of Allegiance, in a line-up of youngsters with right hands held high toward the flag each morning before it was reverently raised. And the sweet sound of children singing from the heart the many grand old anthems.

Then there was the genuine excitement that came with every holiday from Valentine's Day to Christmas. Nothing, except Christmas Eve, could create more magic than our school program. Weeks of decorating and practicing plays, monologues, pantomimes, singing, all in costume. Until finally that memorable night of the year arrived, when through eyes of wonder, the schoolroom turned into a magnificent Broadway Theatre. Packed from wall to wall with spirited parents, tots, and neighbors. The stage was concealed behind curtains drawn across the front of the room in homespun fashion. And partitioned at each end were the dressing rooms where small performers anxiously awaited their turn. After the program, children gleefully exchanged the name-drawn gifts under the tree. And passed around to each in the audience, brown bags of candy and nuts, and bright red apples out of wooden crates. The delightful, mysterious feeling of Christmas garnished one and all and everything, and left its curious footprints.

And never to forget, were the friendly visits to and from neighbors and relatives, where 'old' folks chatted while kids laughed and played mischievously. Swinging back and forth on the ropes in the hayloft, leaping and landing in the sweet-smelling stacks of hay, at least that's what you aimed for. "Anti" over the roof; Hide and Seek; riding clumsy work-horses, cows, or giant squealing pigs; and endless other capers.

Every Sunday I'd sit next to Mom in the little white country church. I remember the faint scent of her perfume, greetings from all the warm and familiar faces, and day-dreaming an enjoyable passing of the hour. Stopping by Grandpa's house afterward, where occasionally he gave me a nickel or a peppermint from the old desk drawer. The cuddly hugs and twinkling brown eyes of my aunt who lived there. Frolicking with the cousins. The pleasant mixed aroma of coffee brewing, fresh-baked sunbockles, lefsa, or other Norwegian delicacies, and tobacco smoke drifting from the room where men gathered for farm talk and witty tales.

Family picnics at the surrounding lakes were also a common merriment, mostly when out-of-town kin folks paid a visit. I recall the lovely classic strains in the open air of an uncle's violin and auntie's mandolin, their perfect blend of voices. And now and then everyone sang together.

It was truly a wonderful life. The fondest kind of place to grow up. And heaven to any child's imagination.

Though the whole story of that time (filled with gentleness and clarity) would take forever to tell."

HOW COULD ANYTHING GO WRONG?

Sadly, there are no guarantees... I had come from what appeared to be the best of families. Not without error, but their intentions were all of the most honorable kind. At age fourteen I was sent to a religious boarding school in Minnesota, too far away for more than one annual homecoming during the school year—the Christmas holidays. There is no question in my mind that the decision was made for all the right reasons. There was no way of knowing the outcome. Back in those days it seemed like many people didn't know how they felt about certain things, much less talked about them. Maybe not altogether a bad trend, in the sense that nowadays we have talked our way into a worse dilemma that has lessened the value of words. In any case, the school had apparently worked well for everyone else. My mother, her seven siblings, my cousins, my brother. A family tradition and considered a privilege.

For me it was an earth-shattering experience that would indeed affect the rest of my life. The homesickness was devastating for the first few months, as though all my close ties of home and security were severed in one great blast. Being the only school of its kind, many of the students were from the big cities of the East coast, the West coast and elsewhere in between. Out of this vast diversity were the more cultured, fashionable, and powerful rulers of the roost, who in the beginning led me to believe I was a nobody, by many tactics not in line with Christian values, as was often the case in the austerity of the faculty also. My concept of God became that of a mean guy who was out to get me. I knew nothing of popularity or peer pressure. From where I came, kids were pretty much all the same. A childish fight now and then, and by the next day it was all over. If apologies were in order they were given. But unlike back home, this was a confounding sort of game that (for one thing) aimed to decide, from an unjustified outward perspective, who was, or was not a "christian". The harder I tried to follow the rules for acceptance, the more I failed, and eventually took my place with the rebels. At least they seemed more real. The mischievous uptown rendezvous, scaling the fire escape after hours from our 4th floor rooms. Puffing cigarettes in cloudy gas station lavatories. The first movie I ever saw was OKLAHOMA. A delightful experience, though strictly against the rules. THE RULES—they were rigid, banning the worldly sinful pleasures of movies, dancing, makeup, et cetera…, of which I became more and more curious towards, until I began questioning most everything I'd been raised to believe. My high school years were confused and rebellious ones.

A year after graduation, my mother died of cancer, preceded by a brief period of diagnosis and apparent illness. Before high school I felt very close to Mom. The greatest person in the world. The epitome of a truly honorable lady. In four years we had become strangers. I knew I had disappointed her, but I didn't know how to change it. Neither did anyone else, other than shame and blame that only made the conflicts worse.

A short time afterward, I left home and in all respects, closed the door on everything in the past. I would start a brand new life, a good life. It even worked for awhile. I grew to love Los Angeles. The beaches, the mountains, the freedom, the excitement of the night-life and never-ending city in the glow of youthful adventure. Nothing at all reminded me of home, except maybe some of the imaginative dreams I'd had back on the little farm, then so remote as though it were another lifetime.

However, accompanying this new-found freedom was often the feeling of being lost. A yearning to go **home**, yet where and what that meant anymore, I did not know. As though at some point long before, it suddenly vanished. Not until many heartbreaks later, did I knowingly begin the painful search for the 'pebbles' to lead the way back. And that was my time of introduction to an endless road of baffling experiences in the "recovery systems" which included various church affiliations often worsening the confusion. Later on this same hopeless frustration would be validated by the plight of numerous other suffering souls. Therapy became a feeling in one sense of *"the blind leading the blind"*. And likewise these lengthy perplexing methods that are supposed to bring healing but all too often are not working—still prevail. **Yet in all fairness**, many of these "systems" may very well be effective for those experiencing depression over recent obvious traumatic events, providing they do not have a history of deep-seated, on-going problems. Besides, there are exceptions to every rule.

It now seems that the details of most people's descending courses, known by many names and behaviors, are not nearly as important as the common state they all share of being **LOST**/disconnected from their original selves. **How did they come to be lost?** Not theologically lost, but what happened way back when—that point in time when the lights went out? And the defenses of survival took over? Furthermore, the initial suffering itself may be equally devastating in most troubled souls, no matter what indicates the outward appearance. Everything after that, is simply the conglomeration of results of being lost. The trouble is, **we can't see it,** because we have been disconnected from the light that was once there in all of us. So the masquerades go on with disparate faces, outcomes, and degrees of severity... until we find that moment when honest reasoning disappeared—the heart of the problem that **must** be healed, before **real** life-change can happen. However, seldom will any of this be effective (**because of the very nature of the disease**) without the person being completely removed from the toxicity of their environment until the healing takes place, and is then given enough time to become rooted and grow in a thriving atmosphere designed for total recovery.

It seems so simple. How do we miss it? Probably because **wisdom forever presents itself in simple truth**. We've looked largely to the complex, long drawn out, inconclusive... methods, that often come in parcels of an hour a week, just enough to be left hanging in frustration over the puzzle 'til next time, as the weeks turn into years. While the afflicted are waiting, or have given up waiting (even though not consciously) for something quite the opposite. Their basic need is to plug back into the Power, reconnect to the original self—which (upon happening) they <u>will</u> recognize it as a familiar state of being, **because it is the common ground (grounding) of the whole human race.** Something, deep within everyone, knows this reality that is called by many names—the god in us, the child, the soul, the source of life, the power of Love... we can't run away from it. The bible characterizes it as such, *"Where can I flee from the presence of your spirit? Even when I make my bed in hell, you are there...."* It

<u>will not</u> be separated from us—EVER, for as long as we live. Only in the "adult mind" interpretations of this, do we get tangled up in disagreement.

In my case again, at age fourteen I was terrified to be so far away from my mother and home. If every other student in the school was ready for that great transition, I WAS NOT! The pain was unbearable. Thus began my unskilled journey to survive, driven by all that I could not understand, no different than the beginning of every other disconnected person's story. The main difference is where or how far we allow that pain to carry us, which seems to have a great deal to do with our backgrounds. For me it was not that apparent on the surface. I learned to be a good actress, when there didn't seem to be another way. Pretend that everything was OK. But inside I was as torn and broken as many of the most obvious lost souls.

Until I discovered that the **homecoming** was not necessarily any particular place nor people, but the reconnection to myself, to the time when I was still whole (all in one piece), when things were instinctively clear even without being told. Although I knew by then I was one of the lucky ones, in spite of having wasted much time and effort trying to find **THE** fault within my fourteen-year upbringing, under the persuasion of many counselors who lacked discernment. And not to say there were no imperfections in those early years, but I finally began to see it as the part of my life I needed most to embrace.

As I look back, it seems clear that I have gleaned the greatest part of my strong beliefs from childhood. The river I've drawn from over and over, in the worst of times, yet never diminished. Now as an 'older' adult, these memories seem to weave in and out of everything I've experienced and come to believe since then. Propelling, as it were, a tremendous passion, first of all, toward the neglect and/or ignorance that continues to exist toward human suffering in a land so blessed with the means to turn it around.

Nevertheless, above all I hold with conviction a vision that could in due time change this course, one that would yield **real healing** to all kinds of desperate souls everywhere. The most significant reason for the certainty is that I have been there, in the 'systems', where multitudes still tread. I know the hopelessness they feel. Perhaps sometimes God allows us to wander in the wilderness to gain personal understanding of the plight of others, so it may lead to a higher good. Assuredly, everything I ever dreamed of or needed to restore my own soul, including all I couldn't find elsewhere (no stone unturned), has finally come together in the framework of this vision. That alone is a miracle. The next is yet to come. And until my time on earth is over, my foremost aspiration is to play a part in its reality.

Meanwhile, the reality of the civilized world remains increasingly surrounded by forces of evil, as the **cause** goes pitifully unattended. **Hopelessness is the chief breeding ground for evil**. And from that infestation come the predators who lie waiting in shadows to threaten one and all—even our homes are no longer safe. While other masses simply suffer. And nations grow weary of wrestling with the turmoil. Our backs are at the sea! **We are at the mercy of a miracle!** First, the miracle of acknowledgement instead of denial. There must be a willingness to **drag it ALL out of the closet** and address it humbly and honestly for the monster we have allowed it to become. Only then are we ready to attack the problem. Replace the flimsy ideology and methods with **uncommon wisdom** championed by stamina to rid this ominous epidemic. Turn our habitual impatience into

something constructive, whereby recovery should take months, not years, a lifetime, or never. Achieve success instead of failure in the crucial issue of **Mental Illness**, which belongs at the top of our priorities. Not another battle to be fought, but a condition to overcome—one by one, as they multiply to great numbers, never ending, of restored individuals... Yet here again, **America** must lead this band of warriors as they march to a different drum, to a new, enlightened realization of the road to Peace. Concession to follow the order, *"Cast the nets on the other side"*, will be to reap the boundless rewards by engagement in an all-out mission:
   OPERATION SOUL RECOVERY...

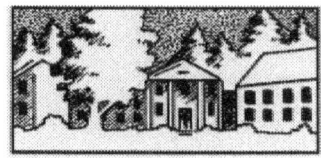

AFTERWORD

FROM A COMPOSITION OF BLANK VERSE, WRITTEN IN 1993

"Wake up you sleeping giants! God's most notable creation!
And listen to the One who walked the earth, spoke of Truth,
And never turned His back on any pain or sickness.
He was not some sanctimonious phantom, He was real.
Why else would all those rugged pioneers, our forefathers,
Have built this nation on His rock?
We've forgotten.
Our pious prayers won't save us.
The gospel without arms and legs is useless.
What did He mean if not exactly what He said?
He could be counted on for certain.
In sight of all His miracles, He left us with these final words,
'Even greater things than these can you do when I'm gone,
If you will just BELIEVE.'
Where are the limits after that?
Moreover what would **still** be closer to His heart,
Than healing human pain?
There is no need nor justice, to die these cruel deaths,
When Someone did it for us long ago.
The problem is we can't conceive of anyone so REAL.
It's foreign to the grownup mind, and more so as time passes.

We are blind and deaf and senseless,
Until we find that awesome child again,
Who holds the keys to Love and Faith and Miracles—
   TO LIFE!
What other part of us would dare to dream great dreams and then,
BELIEVE them into substance?"

Writing a book can often be a form of healing in itself, to find out more of who we are. But ultimately we have something to say that can no longer be confined only within ourselves. If it were not for countless mentors spreading their gospels of confidence that, *"Sometimes God uses imperfect, ordinary people to bring about His extraordinary plans"*, I wouldn't have the courage to carry this heartfelt exposition into the chill of the marketplace. But on that note I will..., and will remain forever grateful to all the inspiring believers who challenge the expression of our visions, dreams and voices, borne from the **Soul.** For in that **Place**, beyond limited thoughts, lie the answers to every problem on earth, including the healing of **mental illness**...

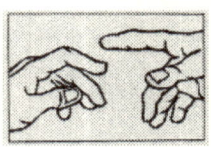

THE END

www.ingramcontent.com/pod-product-compliance
Lightning Source LLC
Chambersburg PA
CBHW030906180526
45163CB00004B/1731